Sweet Alternatives

Exploring Healthy Sugar Substitutes

PUBLISHED BY: Ditya Zulkarnain

Table of Contents:

Introduction

- **Why Choose Healthy Sugar Substitutes?**

In an era where health consciousness is on the rise, the choices we make about what we consume have profound implications for our well-being. One of the most significant dietary shifts in recent years has been the reconsideration of sugar and its alternatives. As concerns over the health impacts of excessive sugar consumption grow, more and more individuals are seeking healthier options to satisfy their sweet tooth without compromising their health.

The book " Sweet Alternatives: Exploring Healthy Sugar Substitutes " delves into this timely and pressing topic, offering readers a comprehensive guide to understanding and selecting the best alternatives to refined sugar. Authored by experts in nutrition and wellness, this book goes beyond mere substitution, exploring the science behind sugar's effects on the body and the benefits of choosing healthier alternatives.

Through meticulous research and practical insights, this book equips readers with the knowledge they need to make informed decisions about their sugar intake. From natural sweeteners like stevia and monk fruit to sugar alcohols and other innovative substitutes, each option is carefully examined for its nutritional profile, taste, and culinary applications.

Moreover, "Why Choose Healthy Sugar Substitutes?" addresses common misconceptions about sugar substitutes, providing clarity on their safety, effectiveness, and suitability for various dietary needs, including those with diabetes or weight management goals.

Whether you're looking to reduce sugar for health reasons, manage a medical condition, or simply adopt a more balanced diet, this book serves as your essential companion. It empowers you to navigate the complex landscape of sweeteners confidently, ensuring that every choice you make contributes positively to your overall health and well-being.

- **Overview of Common Sugar Substitutes**

In today's health-conscious world, the quest for alternatives to traditional sugar has become increasingly important. As more individuals strive to reduce their sugar intake for various health reasons, the market for sugar substitutes has expanded rapidly, offering a plethora of options. Understanding these alternatives is key to making informed choices that promote both health and enjoyment in our diets.

From natural sweeteners like honey, maple syrup, and agave nectar to non-nutritive sweeteners such as stevia, aspartame, and saccharin, each substitute is meticulously scrutinized for its taste, nutritional properties, and suitability for different culinary applications. The book also delves into sugar alcohols like xylitol and erythritol, explaining their benefits and potential drawbacks.

Beyond merely listing substitutes, this book provides readers with a deeper understanding of the science behind these alternatives. It explores how each substitute interacts with the body, addressing concerns about impact on blood sugar levels, dental health, and overall well-being. Moreover, the book discusses the regulatory landscape governing sugar substitutes, ensuring readers are informed about safety and usage guidelines.

Whether you're a health-conscious consumer, a culinary enthusiast, or a healthcare professional seeking reliable information, "Sweet Alternatives: Exploring Healthy Sugar Substitutes" serves as an indispensable resource. It equips you with the knowledge needed to navigate the complex world of sweeteners confidently, empowering you to make choices that align with your health goals and dietary preferences.

Natural Alternatives

1. Stevia: Nature's Sweet Leaf

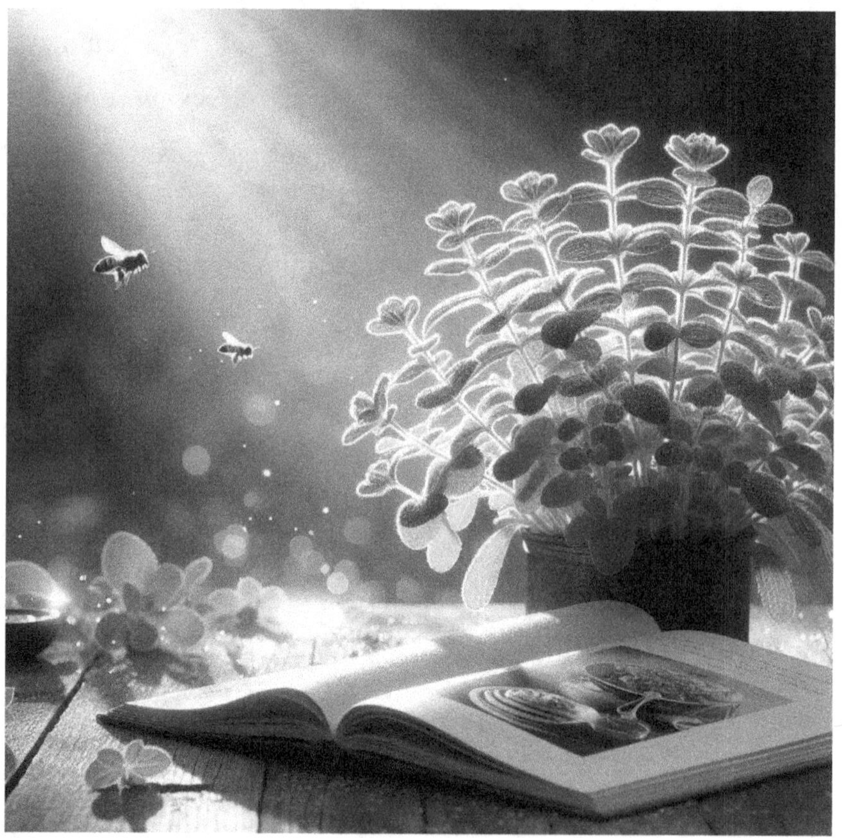

In the quest for healthier eating habits, stevia has emerged as a natural alternative to traditional sugar. Known as "Nature's Sweet Leaf," stevia not only offers sweetness but also brings numerous health benefits without the drawbacks of calories or negative impacts on blood sugar levels. This article delves into the origins, cultivation, scientific aspects, culinary uses, health benefits, and increasing popularity of stevia.

Origins and Cultivation:

Stevia, scientifically known as Stevia rebaudiana, is native to South America, where it has been used for centuries by indigenous tribes for its sweetening properties. The plant thrives in tropical and subtropical regions and is now cultivated in several countries worldwide, including Paraguay, Brazil, China, and Japan. Stevia is primarily grown for its leaves, which contain natural sweet compounds known as steviol glycosides.

Science Behind its Low-Calorie Sweetness:

The sweetness of stevia comes from steviol glycosides, particularly stevioside and rebaudioside A, which are several hundred times sweeter than sucrose (table sugar) on a per weight basis. Despite their intense sweetness, these compounds are non-caloric and do not raise blood glucose levels, making stevia an attractive option for diabetics and those watching their caloric intake.

Benefits in Cooking, Baking, and Beverages:

Stevia is versatile and can be used in various culinary applications. In cooking and baking, stevia extracts or powdered forms can replace sugar in recipes with a much smaller quantity due to its potency. It can be used in both hot and cold beverages, providing sweetness without the need for added sugars or artificial sweeteners. Stevia blends seamlessly into desserts, sauces, and even savory dishes, offering a guilt-free way to satisfy sweet cravings.

Impact on Health:

One of the most significant advantages of stevia is its potential health benefits. Unlike sugar, which contributes to weight gain, tooth decay, and adverse effects on metabolism, stevia offers sweetness without these drawbacks. It does not promote dental cavities and does not affect insulin levels, making it suitable for individuals with diabetes or those on low-calorie diets. Research also suggests potential benefits for managing hypertension and inflammation, although more studies are needed to confirm these effects conclusively.

Growing Popularity:

As consumers become increasingly health-conscious and aware of the detrimental effects of excessive sugar consumption, natural alternatives like stevia are gaining popularity. Stevia is now a common ingredient in many food products marketed as "sugar-free" or "low-sugar," ranging from beverages to snacks and desserts. Its availability in various forms, including liquid extracts and dissolvable tablets, has made it convenient for consumers to incorporate into their daily routines.

As the demand for natural and healthier alternatives grows, stevia stands out as a beacon of sweetness in a world increasingly mindful of dietary choices and their impact on well-being.

2. Monk Fruit: The Miracle Fruit

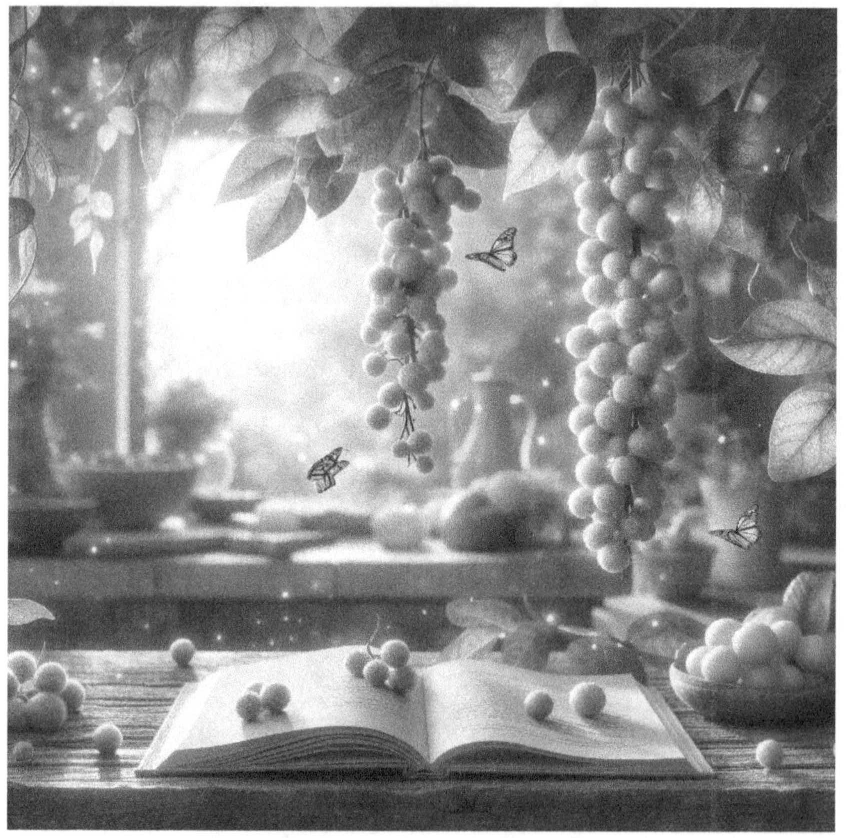

In the realm of natural sweeteners, monk fruit has gained prominence as "The Miracle Fruit" for its intense sweetness without the calories or adverse health effects associated with sugar. This article explores the origins, cultivation, scientific basis of its low-calorie sweetness, benefits in culinary uses, impact on health, and its increasing popularity among consumers seeking natural alternatives to refined sugars.

Origins and Cultivation:

Monk fruit, also known as *Luo Han Guo*, is native to the mountainous regions of Southern China and Northern Thailand. Historically, it has been cultivated by Buddhist monks, hence the name "monk fruit." The fruit itself is small, round, and resembles a melon, but its sweetness primarily comes from compounds called mogrosides found in its flesh and seeds.

Cultivation of monk fruit involves careful nurturing in specific climatic conditions, often in mountainous areas with well-drained soil. It is a perennial vine that requires a warm climate with adequate rainfall for optimal growth.

Science Behind its Low-Calorie Sweetness:

The sweetness of monk fruit is attributed to mogrosides, particularly mogroside V, which is significantly sweeter than sugar but does not contribute calories or carbohydrates to the diet. These compounds are also non-glycemic and do not affect blood sugar levels, making monk fruit an ideal sweetener for individuals with diabetes or those following a low-carbohydrate diet.

Unlike some other sweeteners, monk fruit extract does not have a bitter aftertaste, which enhances its appeal as a natural sugar substitute.

Benefits in Cooking, Baking, and Beverages:

Monk fruit extract is highly concentrated, requiring only a small amount to achieve the desired sweetness in recipes. It blends well in both hot and cold beverages, such as teas, coffees, and smoothies, without altering their flavor profile. In baking and cooking, monk fruit sweetener can replace sugar in a 1:1 ratio in most recipes, providing sweetness without the excess calories.

Due to its heat stability, monk fruit extract can withstand cooking temperatures, making it suitable for use in a wide range of culinary applications, including desserts, sauces, and marinades.

Impact on Health:

The health benefits of monk fruit extend beyond its low-calorie sweetness. It does not contribute to tooth decay, making it tooth-friendly compared to sugar. Its non-glycemic nature means it does not cause spikes in blood sugar levels, offering a safe alternative for those managing diabetes or insulin resistance.

Additionally, monk fruit extract contains antioxidants, which may help combat oxidative stress and inflammation in the body. Some studies suggest potential benefits for respiratory health and immune function, although more research is needed to fully understand these effects.

Growing Popularity:

As awareness of the negative effects of sugar consumption grows, consumers are increasingly turning to natural alternatives like monk fruit. Its zero-calorie, non-glycemic properties make it appealing to health-conscious individuals seeking to reduce their sugar intake without sacrificing sweetness. Monk fruit sweeteners are now widely available in various forms, including liquid extracts, powders, and blends with other natural sweeteners.

The popularity of monk fruit is also evident in its incorporation into a variety of commercial products marketed as "sugar-free" or "no added sugar," ranging from beverages to snacks and desserts. Its versatility and natural origin have contributed to its rapid adoption in the food and beverage industry.

As the demand for natural sweeteners continues to rise, monk fruit stands out for its ability to provide sweetness without the drawbacks of calories or blood sugar spikes, making it a valuable addition to the pantry for those prioritizing both taste and health.

3. Raw Honey: Balancing Sweetness and Health Benefits

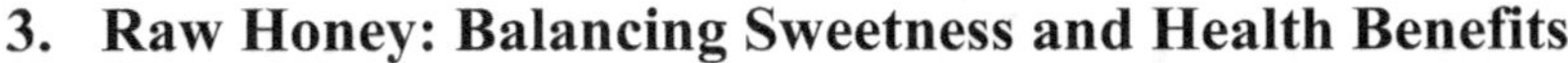

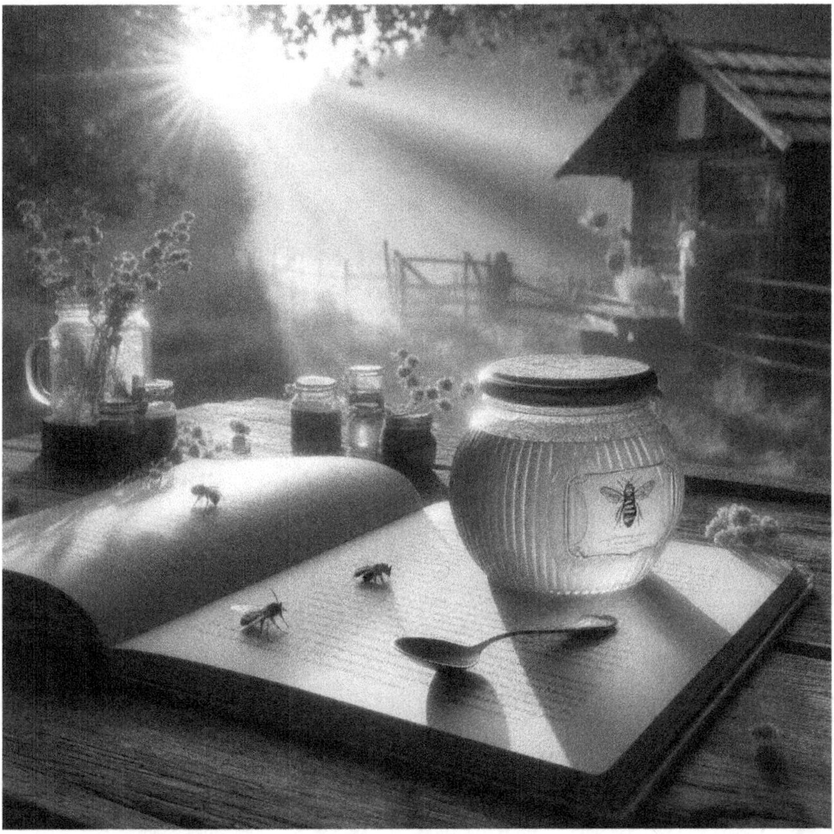

Raw honey has long been cherished not only for its natural sweetness but also for its myriad health benefits, making it a favored alternative to refined sugars. This article delves into the origins, cultivation, scientific aspects of its sweetness, benefits in culinary applications, impact on health, and its increasing popularity among health-conscious consumers.

Origins and Cultivation:

Honey is as ancient as human history itself, with evidence of its consumption dating back thousands of years. Bees produce honey from the nectar of flowers through a process of regurgitation and evaporation. The exact flavor and composition of honey vary depending on the types of flowers visited by the bees. Different floral sources result in variations such as clover honey, wildflower honey, or acacia honey.

Cultivation of honey involves beekeeping, where beekeepers maintain hives and facilitate the collection of honeycomb frames filled with honey. These frames are harvested, and honey is extracted and processed minimally to retain its natural properties.

Science Behind its Sweetness:

The sweetness of honey primarily comes from its composition of sugars, predominantly glucose and fructose, although the exact ratio can vary slightly depending on floral sources. The unique blend of sugars gives honey its distinct taste and sweetness level, which can range from mild to intensely sweet.

Despite its sweetness, raw honey is considered a low-glycemic index food, meaning it does not cause a rapid spike in blood sugar levels compared to refined sugars. This makes it a preferable option for individuals managing their blood sugar levels, although moderation is still advised due to its calorie content.

Benefits in Cooking, Baking, and Beverages:

Raw honey is celebrated in culinary circles for its versatility. It can be used as a natural sweetener in various dishes, from breakfast oats to salad dressings and marinades. In baking, honey adds moisture and depth of flavor to cakes, bread, and cookies, often reducing the need for additional sweeteners or fats. Its ability to caramelize when heated makes it ideal for glazes and sauces.

In beverages, raw honey dissolves easily in both hot and cold liquids, enhancing teas, smoothies, and cocktails with its distinct sweetness and flavor profile. It can also be used to sweeten homemade syrups and lemonades naturally.

Impact on Health:

Beyond its role as a sweetener, raw honey boasts numerous health benefits. It is rich in antioxidants, vitamins, and minerals, including enzymes and amino acids that contribute to its nutritional profile. These antioxidants help protect the body from oxidative stress and inflammation, potentially reducing the risk of chronic diseases.

Raw honey is also renowned for its antimicrobial properties, which can help support immune function and promote wound healing when applied topically. However, it is important to note that these benefits are most pronounced in raw honey, as heating or processing can degrade its nutritional value.

Growing Popularity:

As consumers become more health-conscious and seek natural alternatives to refined sugars, raw honey has experienced a resurgence in popularity. Its wholesome image as a minimally processed, natural sweetener aligns with contemporary dietary trends focused on whole foods and sustainability.

Raw honey's availability in local markets, farmers' markets, and specialty stores underscores its appeal as a locally sourced product with potential benefits for both personal health and environmental sustainability. Its versatility in cooking and baking applications further enhances its attractiveness as a pantry staple for health-conscious households.

Whether enjoyed drizzled over yogurt, stirred into tea, or used to glaze meats, raw honey embodies the balance of sweetness and nutritional value that resonates with today's wellness-focused consumers. As awareness grows of its potential health benefits and culinary uses, raw honey remains a timeless staple, fostering a connection between nature's bounty and our daily enjoyment of food

.

4. Maple Syrup: More Than Just Pancakes

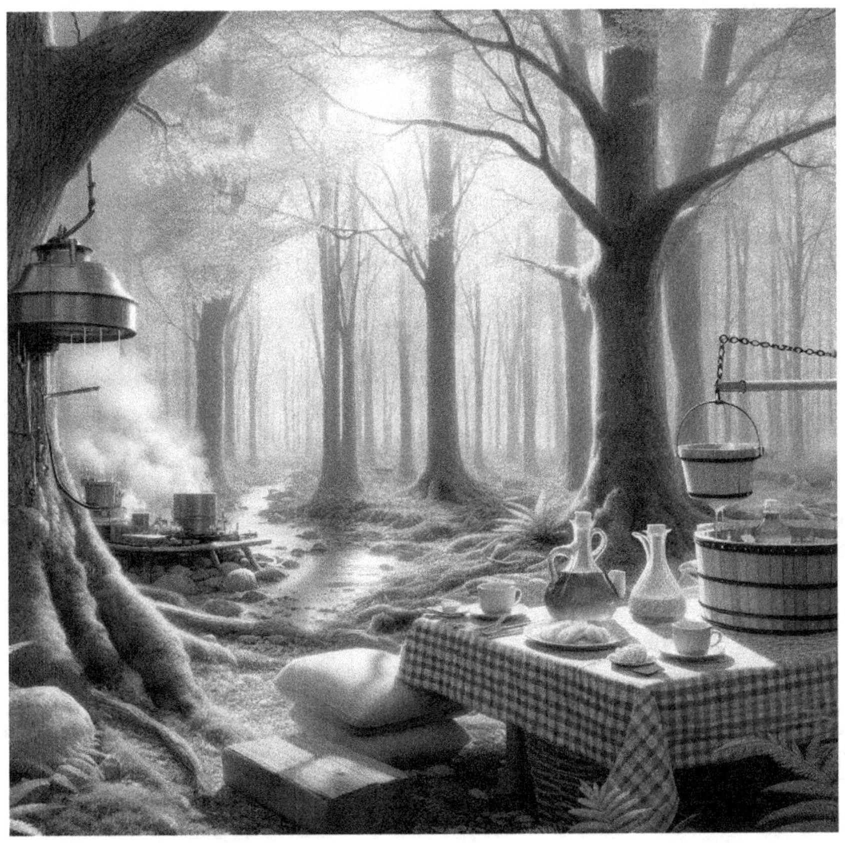

Maple syrup is celebrated not only for its rich, distinctive flavor but also for its status as a natural sweetener that offers several health benefits. This article explores the origins, cultivation, scientific aspects of its sweetness, benefits in culinary uses, impact on health, and its growing popularity among health-conscious consumers seeking natural alternatives to refined sugars.

Origins and Cultivation:

Maple syrup is derived from the sap of sugar maple trees (*Acer saccharum*), which are primarily found in the northeastern United States and Canada. The process of tapping maple trees for sap and boiling it down to concentrate the sugars into syrup has been practiced by Indigenous peoples for centuries and continues today with modern methods.

During early spring, as temperatures fluctuate between freezing at night and thawing during the day, the sap flows through taps drilled into the maple trees. This sap is then collected and boiled down in sugarhouses to remove excess water, resulting in the thick, sweet syrup known for its characteristic maple flavor.

Science Behind its Low-Calorie Sweetness:

Maple syrup's sweetness comes primarily from sucrose, with smaller amounts of glucose and fructose. Despite its sweet taste, maple syrup has a lower glycemic index compared to refined sugars, meaning it causes a slower rise in blood sugar levels. This property makes it a preferred sweetener for those monitoring their blood glucose levels or following a low-glycemic diet.

Additionally, maple syrup contains various antioxidants and minerals, such as manganese and zinc, which contribute to its nutritional value and potential health benefits.

Benefits in Cooking, Baking, and Beverages:

Maple syrup is renowned for its versatility in culinary applications. It adds a distinct sweetness and depth of flavor to a wide range of dishes, from breakfast favorites like pancakes and waffles to savory dishes like roasted vegetables and glazes for meats. In baking, maple syrup can replace granulated sugar in recipes, adding moisture and a rich flavor profile to cakes, cookies, and muffins.

In beverages, maple syrup can be used to sweeten teas, coffees, and smoothies, offering a natural alternative to processed sugars or artificial sweeteners. Its ability to dissolve easily makes it convenient for use in both hot and cold drinks.

Impact on Health:

Beyond its role as a sweetener, maple syrup offers several health benefits. It contains antioxidants, which help combat oxidative stress and inflammation in the body, potentially reducing the risk of chronic diseases. The presence of minerals like manganese supports enzyme function and metabolism, while zinc contributes to immune health and wound healing.

Maple syrup also boasts a unique flavor profile that enhances food satisfaction, potentially reducing the overall consumption of added sugars and promoting mindful eating habits.

Growing Popularity:

As consumers increasingly prioritize natural and minimally processed foods, maple syrup has gained popularity as a healthier alternative to refined sugars and artificial sweeteners. Its wholesome image as a product of nature, harvested from maple trees and minimally processed into syrup, resonates with consumers seeking sustainable and nutritious food choices.

The availability of maple syrup in various grades, from darker, robust flavors to lighter, delicate options, allows consumers to choose based on their flavor preferences and culinary needs. Its integration into a diverse array of products, including granola bars, sauces, and salad dressings, underscores its versatility and widespread appeal.

As awareness grows of its antioxidant content, lower glycemic index, and versatility in culinary applications, maple syrup remains a staple in kitchens worldwide. Its ability to enhance dishes from breakfast to dinner, coupled with its status as a sustainable and natural product, solidifies maple syrup's place as a beloved sweetener for those seeking to balance taste with health-conscious choices.

Artificial Sweeteners

1. Aspartame: Understanding the Controversy

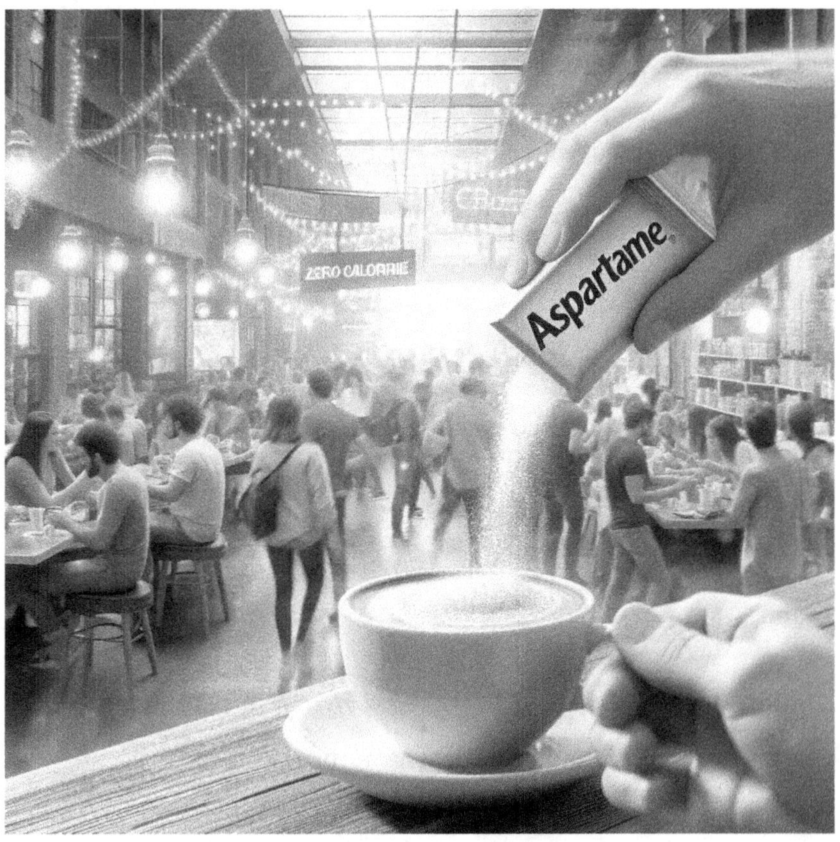

The debate surrounding aspartame, an artificial sweetener widely used in beverages and foods, reflects contrasting perceptions on health, taste, and convenience compared to natural sugar. Understanding both sides involves examining its benefits, controversies, and scientific perspectives.

Benefits of Aspartame:

1. Caloric Reduction:

Aspartame provides sweetness without the caloric load of sugar, making it attractive for those seeking to reduce calorie intake or manage weight.

2. Diabetes Management:

Aspartame does not raise blood sugar levels, making it suitable for people with diabetes who need to monitor their glucose intake.

3. Dental Health:

Unlike sugar, which contributes to tooth decay, aspartame doesn't promote dental caries, benefiting oral health.

Controversies and Concerns:

1. Safety Concerns:

Aspartame has been extensively studied and deemed safe for consumption by regulatory agencies such as the FDA and EFSA. However, some studies and consumer groups raise concerns about potential long-term health effects, including neurological issues and cancer risk, though scientific consensus largely refutes these claims.

2. Taste and Palatability:

While aspartame provides sweetness, some consumers find its taste less satisfying compared to sugar, which can affect product preference and consumption habits.

3. Perception of 'Artificial':

There is a perception among some consumers that artificial sweeteners like aspartame are less natural or healthy compared to sugar, influencing consumer choices based on perceived health risks.

Scientific Insights:

1. Safety Studies:

Numerous studies, including long-term research, support the safety of aspartame within recommended daily intake levels (ADI). The FDA sets ADI limits far below levels shown to cause adverse effects in studies.

2. Health Impacts:

Scientific reviews and meta-analyses generally find no causal link between aspartame consumption and serious health issues like cancer or neurological disorders when consumed within recommended limits.

3. Consumer Preferences:

Preferences for sweeteners can vary widely based on cultural, taste, and health considerations. While some prefer the taste of natural sugars, others opt for artificial sweeteners for health reasons or to manage dietary needs like weight control or diabetes.

Making Informed Choices:

Balanced decision-making involves considering individual health needs, preferences, and scientific consensus:

Health Considerations:

Aspartame can be a safe alternative for reducing calorie intake and managing conditions like diabetes, but individuals should consult ealthcare providers for personalized advice.

Taste and Palatability:

Preferences for sweeteners are subjective, and products using aspartame may differ in taste from those using sugar. Trying different options can help find what suits personal taste preferences.

Regulatory Oversight:

Trusting regulatory agencies' assessments, such as the FDA and EFSA, provides assurance regarding safety within established limits.

In conclusion, the debate over aspartame involves weighing its benefits in calorie reduction and diabetes management against concerns about taste, safety, and perceptions of artificiality. Scientific consensus supports its safety when consumed within recommended limits, but individual preferences and health considerations should guide choices in dietary sweeteners. Understanding these factors empowers consumers to make informed decisions aligned with their health goals and taste preferences.

2. Sucralose: Unveiling the Sweet Truth

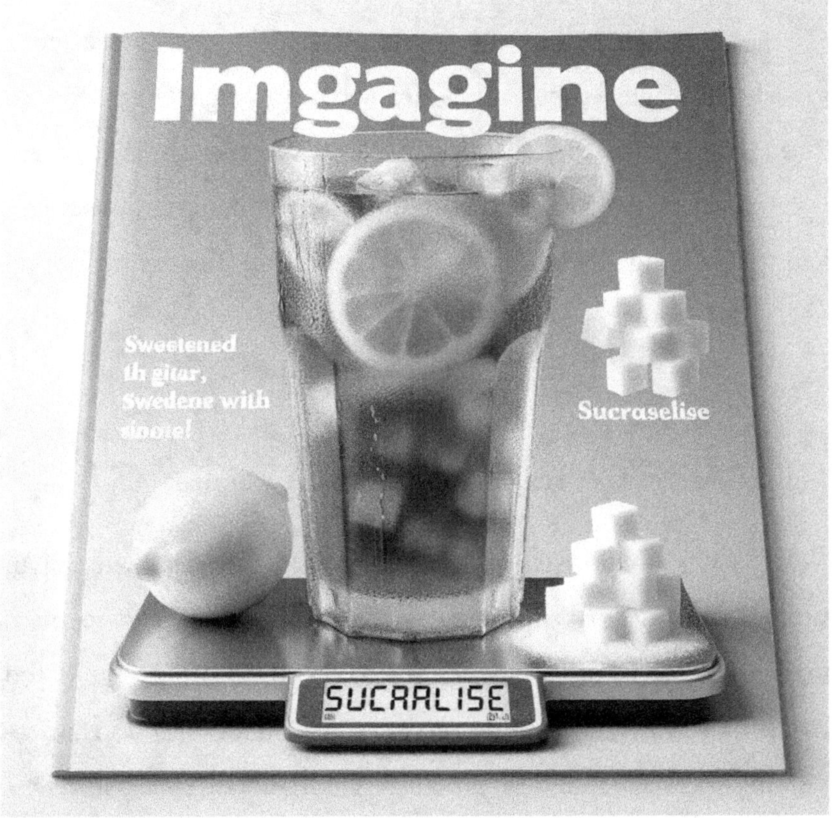

Sucralose has emerged as a popular artificial sweetener renowned for its intense sweetness without the caloric impact of sugar. This book delves into its creation, impact on taste perception, controversies surrounding its safety, and its broad applications in various food and beverage products.

The Science Behind Sucralose

Sucralose was discovered in 1976 by researchers investigating new compounds derived from sugar. It is created through a process that substitutes three chlorine atoms for three hydroxyl groups on a sucrose molecule, enhancing sweetness and preventing metabolism by the body, thus contributing negligible calories to the diet.

Impact on Taste Perception and Dietary Choices

Sucralose is approximately 600 times sweeter than sugar, allowing for minimal usage to achieve desired sweetness in foods and beverages. Its sweetness profile is often considered similar to sugar, making it a popular choice for consumers looking to reduce calorie intake without sacrificing taste. This characteristic has led to its widespread adoption in products marketed as "sugar-free" or "diet."

Controversies and Safety Concerns

Despite its widespread use, sucralose has faced scrutiny regarding its safety. Regulatory agencies like the FDA and EFSA have deemed it safe for human consumption based on extensive scientific research. Studies have consistently shown no evidence of carcinogenicity or adverse health effects when consumed within recommended limits. However, some concerns persist among certain consumer groups and studies that suggest potential impacts on gut microbiota or metabolic responses.

Applications in Food Products

Sucralose's stability under heat makes it suitable for a variety of food products, including baked goods, candies, and beverages. Its ability to withstand high temperatures without losing sweetness has made it a preferred choice for manufacturers seeking to create low-calorie or sugar-free alternatives to traditional sugar-sweetened products.

Consumer Appeal and Preferences

Consumers gravitate towards sucralose for its ability to provide sweetness without the guilt of excess calories or adverse effects on blood sugar levels. Its versatility in applications allows for a wide range of products catering to different dietary needs, including those of individuals managing diabetes or watching their calorie intake.

Making Informed Choices

When considering sweetener options, it's crucial to weigh the scientific consensus on safety against personal preferences and dietary goals. Sucralose offers a viable alternative to sugar for many individuals, providing sweetness without the metabolic impacts associated with sugar consumption. However, as with any food additive, moderation and understanding personal tolerance are key factors in making informed dietary choices.

In conclusion, Sucralose stands as a testament to innovation in food technology, offering a potent alternative to sugar with minimal caloric impact. While controversies exist regarding its safety, regulatory approvals and extensive scientific research generally support its use within *recommended limits*. Understanding sucralose's role in the food industry empowers consumers to navigate their dietary choices effectively, balancing taste preferences with health considerations for a well-rounded approach to nutrition

3. Saccharin: A Journey Through Time and Taste

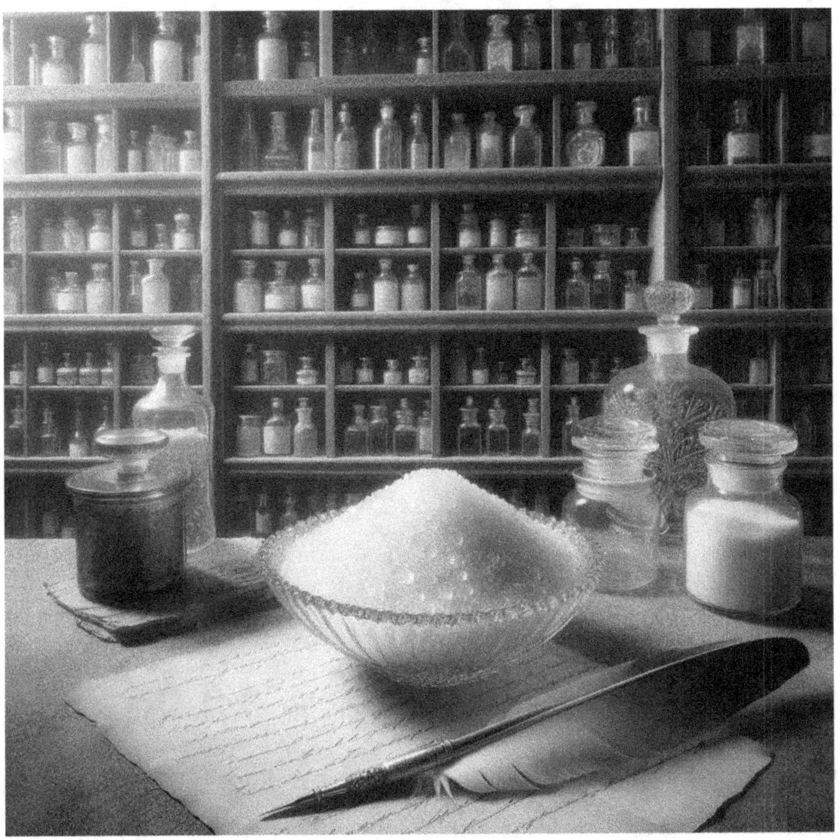

Saccharin, the venerable artificial sweetener, has etched its mark on culinary history, evolving from accidental discovery to widespread use in today's diet-conscious society. This article embarks on a journey through its rich history, explores its impact on health debates, and analyzes its enduring appeal and scientific research.

The Origins and Evolution of Saccharin

Saccharin's story begins in 1879, when chemist Constantin Fahlberg stumbled upon its sweet taste while working in the lab. This accidental discovery sparked a revolution in the sweetener industry, paving the way for saccharin's commercial production and use as a sugar substitute during times of scarcity, including World War I and II.

Reputation and Controversies

Throughout its history, saccharin has weathered controversies surrounding its safety. In the early 20th century, concerns over potential health risks led to its temporary ban in certain countries, though subsequent research and regulatory reviews reinstated its use under strict safety guidelines. Today, saccharin enjoys regulatory approval from agencies like the FDA and EFSA, affirming its safety when consumed within recommended limits.

Enduring Appeal in Modern Society

Saccharin continues to thrive in modern dietary landscapes, valued for its intense sweetness—approximately 300 to 400 times sweeter than sugar—while contributing negligible calories. Its stability under heat makes it ideal for a variety of culinary applications, including beverages, baked goods, and tabletop sweeteners, catering to consumers seeking to manage weight or control sugar intake.

Scientific Insights on Safety and Comparative Benefits

Scientific research supports saccharin's safety profile when used appropriately. Studies have consistently shown no evidence of carcinogenicity or adverse health effects in humans at typical consumption levels. Its advantages over natural sugars include its ability to sweeten without contributing to tooth decay and its suitability for individuals with diabetes due to its negligible impact on blood glucose levels.

Nuanced Perspective on Incorporating Saccharin

Consumers considering saccharin should weigh its benefits, such as calorie reduction and diabetic-friendly properties, against individual taste preferences and health considerations. Like any food additive, moderation is key, and those with specific health concerns should consult healthcare professionals for personalized advice.

In conclusion, Saccharin stands as a testament to human ingenuity and innovation in the quest for healthier dietary alternatives. From its humble beginnings in a laboratory to its integration into everyday foods and beverages, saccharin continues to shape how we sweeten our lives. Armed with scientific understanding and historical context, consumers can make informed choices about incorporating saccharin into their diets, balancing taste preferences with health-conscious decisions for a well-rounded approach to nutrition.

Plant-Based Options

1. Coconut Sugar: A Nutrient-Rich Sweetener

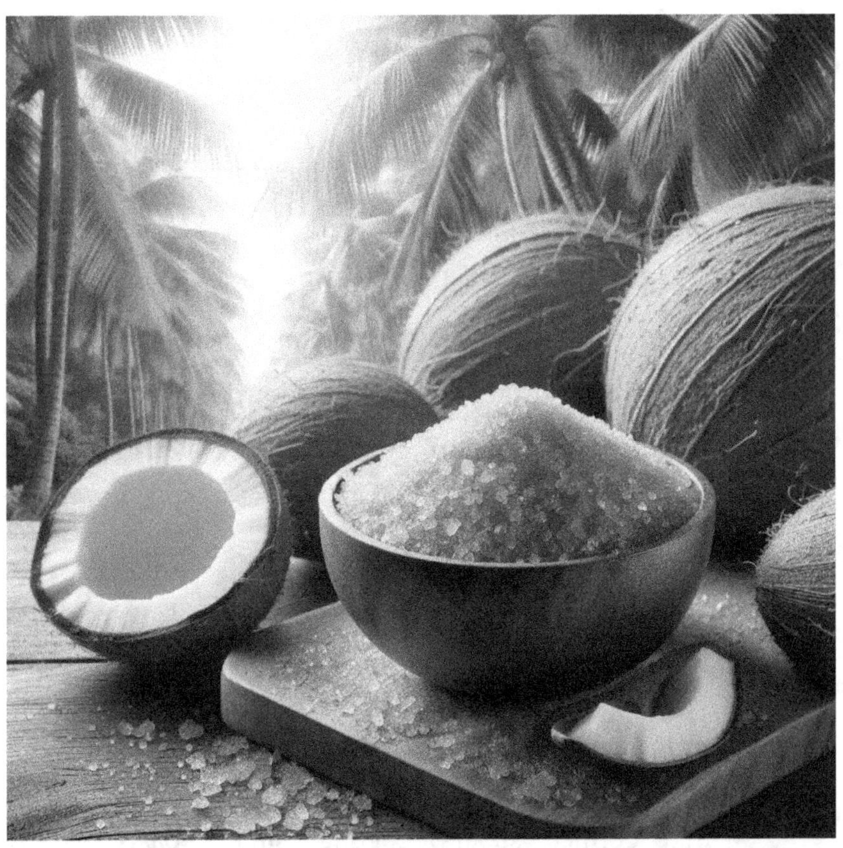

Coconut sugar has surged in popularity as a natural, nutrient-rich alternative to traditional sugars, celebrated for its origins, nutritional profile, and culinary versatility. This book explores its journey from the sap of coconut palm trees to kitchen tables worldwide, emphasizing its sustainable practices, health benefits, and creative culinary applications.

Origins and Sustainable Harvesting

Coconut sugar originates from the sap of coconut palm trees, a process that involves extracting the sap, heating it to evaporate moisture, and finally crystallizing it into granules. This traditional method ensures minimal processing, preserving the natural goodness of the sap without additives or chemicals. The sustainable harvesting of coconut sugar supports local economies and promotes environmental conservation by utilizing renewable coconut palm resources.

Nutritional Riches and Health Benefits

Unlike refined sugars, coconut sugar boasts a rich nutritional profile. It contains essential vitamins such as vitamin C, B vitamins (especially B1, B2, B3, and B6), and minerals like potassium, magnesium, zinc, and iron. Additionally, it is rich in antioxidants such as polyphenols, which help combat oxidative stress in the body. The lower glycemic index of coconut sugar (compared to table sugar) means it causes a slower rise in blood sugar levels, making it a preferred choice for individuals managing diabetes or seeking to stabilize energy levels throughout the day.

Culinary Delights and Creative Uses

Coconut sugar's flavor profile is subtly sweet with a hint of caramel, making it ideal for a variety of culinary applications. It can be used as a 1:1 substitute for white or brown sugar in baking recipes, imparting a unique depth of flavor to cookies, cakes, and muffins. Its ability to dissolve easily makes it suitable for sweetening beverages like coffee, tea, and smoothies, enhancing both taste and nutritional value.

Incorporating Coconut Sugar into Your Diet

For individuals pursuing a balanced and plant-based lifestyle, coconut sugar offers a natural alternative that aligns with health-conscious choices. Its versatility in both sweet and savory dishes encourages exploration in the kitchen, from homemade granola and salad dressings to sauces and marinades. By incorporating coconut sugar mindfully into daily meals, individuals can enjoy its benefits while reducing reliance on highly processed sugars.

Conclusion

Coconut sugar represents more than just a sweetener—it embodies a commitment to health, sustainability, and culinary diversity. Its journey from the tropics to global markets highlights its appeal among health-conscious consumers seeking natural alternatives to refined sugars. By understanding its nutritional benefits, exploring creative recipes, and embracing its sustainable origins, individuals can confidently integrate coconut sugar into their diets, fostering a flavorful and nourishing approach to eating well. Whether enhancing baked goods or beverages, coconut sugar stands as a testament to the rich offerings of nature, inviting all to savor its sweetness in harmony with health and wellness.

2. Date Sugar: Sweetness from the Desert

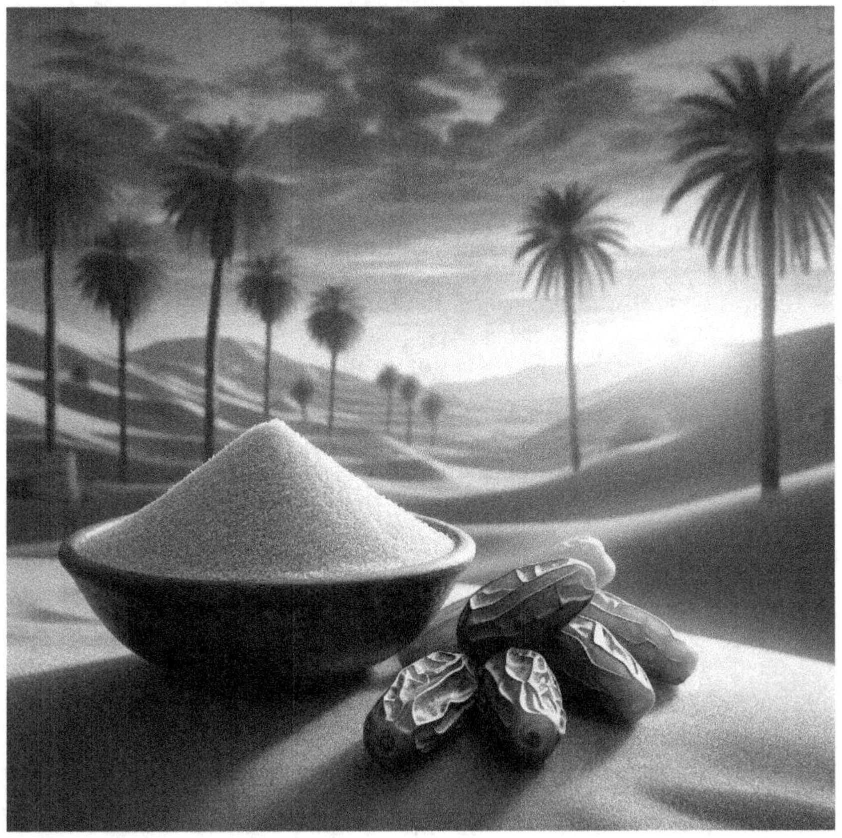

Date sugar, derived from the revered fruit of desert palm trees, offers a journey into both cultural heritage and nutritional richness. This article explores its origins, unique flavor profile, health benefits, and diverse culinary applications, inviting readers to embrace date sugar as a wholesome and sustainable sweetener.

Ancient Origins and Cultural Heritage

Date sugar production dates back centuries, originating in Middle Eastern and North African cultures where dates have been cherished for their sweetness and nutritional value. Traditional methods involve drying dates and grinding them into a fine powder, preserving their natural sweetness and aromatic qualities without additives or processing aids. This ancient practice reflects a deep cultural appreciation for the date palm as a symbol of sustenance and hospitality.

Natural Sweetness and Rich Flavor Profile

Date sugar distinguishes itself with a distinct caramel-like sweetness and robust flavor. Its deep, earthy notes lend a unique depth to dishes, enhancing both sweet and savory recipes. Unlike refined sugars, date sugar retains the fruit's natural sugars, fibers, and trace minerals, offering a more complex and nutrient-dense alternative.

Nutritional Benefits

Rich in dietary fiber, dates support digestive health and contribute to a feeling of fullness. They are also packed with essential vitamins and minerals, including potassium, magnesium, copper, and manganese. These nutrients play vital roles in supporting overall health, from bone strength to energy metabolism. Date sugar's low glycemic index makes it a suitable choice for individuals managing blood sugar levels, providing sustained energy release without the rapid spikes associated with refined sugars.

Culinary Versatility and Innovative Uses

Date sugar's fine texture and intense sweetness make it versatile in culinary applications. It can be used as a 1:1 substitute for brown sugar in baking, imparting a delightful caramel flavor to cookies, cakes, and muffins. It blends seamlessly into beverages like smoothies or tea, adding natural sweetness and nutritional benefits. In savory dishes, date sugar can enhance marinades, sauces, and dressings, offering a hint of sweetness that complements a range of flavors.

Embracing Date Sugar in Your Diet

For health-conscious individuals and those exploring plant-based diets, date sugar presents a wholesome alternative that aligns with sustainable dietary practices. By incorporating date sugar into daily meals, whether in breakfast oats, homemade energy bars, or desserts, individuals can enjoy its rich flavor and nutritional advantages while reducing reliance on processed sugars.

Conclusion

Date sugar stands as a testament to the richness of natural sweetness rooted in cultural heritage and nutritional abundance. From its ancient origins to modern culinary applications, date sugar invites exploration and creativity in the kitchen. By understanding its benefits—nutrient density, low glycemic index, and versatile uses—readers can embrace date sugar as a flavorful and sustainable addition to their dietary repertoire. Whether sweetening baked goods, enhancing beverages, or adding depth to savory dishes, date sugar offers a wholesome alternative that celebrates both taste and health, embodying the essence of a balanced and nourishing lifestyle.

3. Yacon Syrup: The Low-Calorie Sweetener

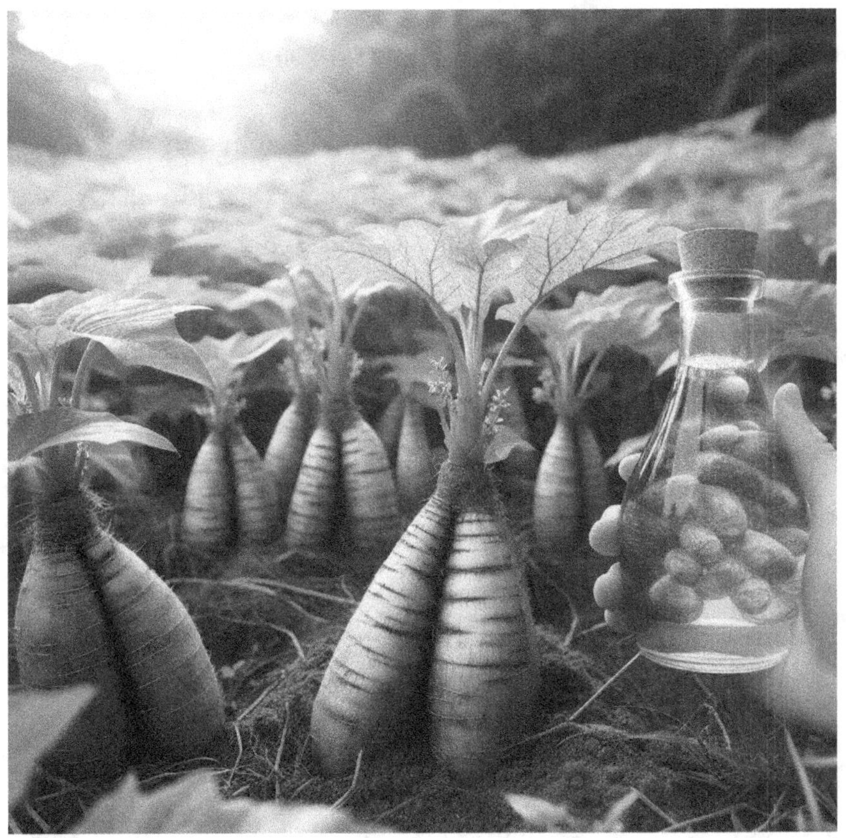

Yacon syrup, derived from the roots of the yacon plant native to South America, offers a fascinating journey into its cultural heritage, health benefits, and culinary delights. This article uncovers the centuries-old history of yacon's use as a natural sweetener, its unique composition, emerging scientific research, and versatile culinary applications.

Cultural Heritage and Centuries-Old Use

Indigenous Andean cultures have long revered yacon for its sweetness and medicinal properties. Traditionally, the roots were consumed raw or in teas for their natural sweetness and digestive benefits. The syrup extraction process involves juicing and concentrating yacon roots, preserving its natural sweetness without the need for extensive processing, aligning with sustainable agricultural practices.

Unique Composition and Health Benefits

Yacon syrup stands out for its high content of fructooligosaccharides (FOS), a type of soluble fiber and prebiotic that passes undigested through the digestive tract, providing sweetness without significantly impacting blood sugar levels. This makes it a preferred choice for individuals managing diabetes or seeking to reduce calorie intake. Moreover, FOS supports gut health by promoting the growth of beneficial bacteria, aiding digestion, and potentially enhancing metabolic health.

Scientific Insights and Emerging Research

Recent studies highlight yacon syrup's potential health benefits beyond its low glycemic index. Research suggests it may help regulate appetite, improve insulin sensitivity, and reduce cholesterol levels. These findings contribute to its growing popularity among health-conscious consumers seeking natural alternatives to refined sugars.

Culinary Versatility and Creative Uses

Yacon syrup's mild, sweet flavor with hints of caramel makes it a versatile ingredient in culinary creations. It can be used as a natural sweetener in beverages like coffee or tea, drizzled over pancakes or yogurt, or incorporated into salad dressings and marinades. Its low calorie content and unique taste profile offer a refreshing twist in both sweet and savory dishes, appealing to those exploring diverse flavors in their diet.

Nutritional Profile and Sustainable Cultivation

Yacon syrup's nutritional profile includes essential minerals such as potassium and phosphorus, along with antioxidants that support overall well-being. Its sustainable cultivation practices, often practiced on small farms in the Andean region, contribute to local economies while preserving traditional agricultural knowledge and biodiversity.

Embracing Yacon Syrup in Your Diet

For individuals seeking to enhance their health-conscious lifestyles, yacon syrup presents a natural, low-calorie alternative to sugar with multifaceted benefits. By incorporating yacon syrup into everyday meals and treats, individuals can enjoy its sweetening properties while supporting gut health and metabolic function. Understanding its cultural significance, nutritional advantages, and culinary versatility empowers readers to make informed choices that promote both personal well-being and sustainable agricultural practices.

Conclusion

Yacon syrup embodies the essence of a natural, health-promoting sweetener rooted in centuries-old traditions and backed by modern scientific research. From its origins in the Andes to its adoption in global cuisine, yacon syrup invites exploration and innovation in the kitchen. By embracing its unique composition, health benefits, and culinary potential, individuals can embark on a flavorful journey that harmonizes taste, nutrition, and sustainability in their dietary choices. Incorporating yacon syrup enriches not only culinary experiences but also supports a balanced approach to wellness, ensuring sweetness with every drop, naturally.

Understanding Glycemic Index

- **Impact of Sugar Substitutes on Blood Sugar Levels**

Sugar substitutes, including both artificial sweeteners and natural alternatives like stevia and monk fruit, have gained popularity as alternatives to regular sugar due to their low-calorie or zero-calorie nature. Understanding their effects on blood sugar regulation, particularly their impact on insulin response, is crucial for individuals managing diabetes or aiming to reduce sugar intake.

Artificial Sweeteners

Artificial sweeteners such as aspartame (Equal), sucralose (Splenda), and saccharin (Sweet'N Low) are synthetic compounds that provide sweetness without calories. These sweeteners are not metabolized like sugar and generally do not raise blood glucose levels. Here's how they affect insulin response:

1. **Insulin Response**: Artificial sweeteners are considered non-nutritive because they are not metabolized for energy. Therefore, they typically do not trigger insulin

release in the same way as sugar does. Studies have shown that artificial sweeteners generally have minimal to no effect on insulin levels.

2. **Benefit for Diabetes Management**: For individuals with diabetes, artificial sweeteners can be beneficial because they provide sweetness without significantly impacting blood sugar levels. They can help satisfy sweet cravings without causing spikes in glucose.

3. **Safety**: Artificial sweeteners are rigorously tested for safety and have been approved by regulatory agencies like the FDA. They are considered safe for most people, including those with diabetes, when consumed within recommended limits.

Natural Alternatives (Stevia and Monk Fruit)

Stevia and monk fruit are natural sweeteners derived from plants. They are often considered more "natural" alternatives to artificial sweeteners and sugar. Here's their impact on blood sugar regulation:

1. **Insulin Response**: Both stevia and monk fruit are low in carbohydrates and do not significantly raise blood glucose levels. They are metabolized differently

compared to sugar and do not typically stimulate insulin secretion.

2. **Benefit for Diabetes Management**: Similar to artificial sweeteners, stevia and monk fruit can be useful for individuals with diabetes as they do not cause spikes in blood sugar levels. They can be used as substitutes for sugar in various foods and beverages.

3. **Safety**: Stevia and monk fruit are generally regarded as safe. Stevia has been approved as a sweetener in many countries, including the US and EU. Monk fruit extract is also widely used as a sweetener and is considered safe when consumed in moderation.

Considerations and Recommendations

- **Individual Variability**: Responses to sugar substitutes can vary among individuals. Some people may experience gastrointestinal discomfort with certain artificial sweeteners or prefer the taste of natural alternatives.

- **Weight Management**: Sugar substitutes can aid in weight management because they provide sweetness without the calories of sugar, which may help reduce overall calorie intake.

- **Long-Term Effects**: While short-term studies generally support the safety of sugar substitutes, the long-term effects of regular consumption are still under investigation. Some studies suggest potential impacts on gut microbiota and metabolic health, but more research is needed.

- **Moderation**: Like any food additive, sugar substitutes should be consumed in moderation. Excessive intake of sweet-tasting substances, even if they do not contain calories, may still influence taste preferences and cravings.

So the conclusion is that Sugar substitutes, both artificial and natural, offer an alternative to regular sugar for individuals who want to manage blood sugar levels, especially for people with diabetes. They generally do not increase blood glucose levels or stimulate insulin secretion as sugar does, making them a valuable tool in diabetes management and sugar reduction strategies. However, individual preference and tolerance should be considered, and moderation is advised to ensure balanced dietary habits. Ongoing research will continue to refine our understanding of its long-term impacts on health.

Baking and Cooking with Substitutes

Tips and Tricks for Successful Sugar Substitutes

In today's culinary landscape, many are exploring alternatives to traditional sugar for various reasons, including health concerns, dietary preferences, or simply experimenting with new flavors. Substituting sugar in baking and cooking requires a nuanced approach to ensure both taste and texture are preserved. Here's a comprehensive guide to help you navigate the world of sugar substitutes effectively.

Understanding Sweeteners

There are numerous sugar substitutes available, each with its own unique properties:

- **Honey**: Adds moisture and subtle floral notes. It's sweeter than sugar, so reduce the amount used and adjust other liquids in the recipe.
- **Maple Syrup**: Offers a rich, caramel-like flavor. It's liquid, so decrease other liquids in the recipe accordingly.
- **Stevia**: A plant-based sweetener that is intensely sweet; a little goes a long way. It doesn't add bulk or moisture,

so recipes may need adjustments to compensate for lost volume.

- **Coconut Sugar**: Has a caramel-like flavor with a lower glycemic index than white sugar. It can generally be substituted 1:1 in recipes.
- **Agave Nectar**: Sweeter than sugar, with a mild flavor. Reduce other liquids in the recipe and monitor baking time as it can cause quicker browning.

Choosing the right substitute depends on the recipe's requirements and your desired flavor profile. Experimentation and tasting throughout the cooking process are key to achieving the best results.

Adjusting Recipes

When substituting sugar, consider these adjustments:

- **Texture**: Sugar contributes to texture in baked goods by creaming with fats and incorporating air. Substitute with a moist ingredient (like applesauce or yogurt) or add an extra egg to maintain texture.
- **Moisture**: Sugar holds moisture in recipes. Substitutes like honey or maple syrup add moisture, while dry sweeteners like stevia may require adding more liquid.

- **Browning**: Sugar caramelizes to create a golden crust. Substitutes like honey or maple syrup may cause quicker browning, so adjust baking temperatures accordingly.

Enhancing Flavor

To enhance flavors when using substitutes:

- **Spices and extracts**: Incorporate cinnamon, vanilla, or citrus zest to amplify flavors.
- **Complementary ingredients**: Use ingredients like nuts, dried fruits, or chocolate to balance flavors and add complexity.

Maintaining Texture

Tips for preserving texture:

- **Hydration**: Use moist substitutes or increase liquid ingredients.
- **Binding**: Add extra eggs or use ingredients like mashed bananas or pumpkin puree to bind ingredients together.

Baking Techniques

Specific techniques for successful baking:

- **Temperature control**: Monitor baking times closely due to variations in caramelization rates.
- **Mixing**: Adjust mixing times to accommodate different textures when using substitutes.

Health Considerations

Considerations when choosing substitutes:

- **Glycemic index**: Some substitutes (e.g., stevia, coconut sugar) have lower glycemic indices than sugar.
- **Calorie content**: While substitutes may offer different calorie profiles, moderation is key.

Practical Applications

Real-life examples and recipes:

- **Cookies**: Use applesauce or mashed bananas in place of sugar for chewy cookies.

- **Cakes**: Replace sugar with honey or maple syrup for moist cakes.
- **Sauces and dressings**: Use stevia or agave nectar in dressings for a touch of sweetness.

Q&A Section

Common reader questions:

- **Can I substitute any sweetener in any recipe?**

  It depends on the recipe and desired outcome. Experimentation is key.

- **How do I prevent my baked goods from becoming too dry when using substitutes?**

  Add moisture-rich ingredients or increase liquids in the recipe.

- **What's the best substitute for achieving a golden crust in baked goods?**

  Honey or maple syrup, but watch for quicker browning.

Substituting sugar in baking and cooking requires understanding the unique properties of each substitute and how they interact with other ingredients. By experimenting with different options and techniques, you can create delicious dishes that meet your dietary preferences and health goals while satisfying your sweet tooth. Happy baking! ^_^

Recipes and Conversion Charts

Substituting sugar in recipes can be both a health-conscious choice and a culinary adventure. Whether you're aiming to reduce calories, manage glycemic index, or explore new flavors, understanding how to effectively use sugar substitutes is key to achieving delicious results. Here's a comprehensive guide to help you navigate recipes and conversion charts when substituting sugar in your culinary creations.

Understanding Sugar Substitutes

1. **Honey**: Offers sweetness with a distinct floral flavor. It's sweeter than sugar, so use less and adjust liquids in recipes.

2. **Maple Syrup**: Adds a rich, caramel-like sweetness. It's liquid, so decrease other liquids in recipes when using it.

3. **Agave Nectar**: Sweeter than sugar with a mild flavor. Reduce other liquids and monitor baking time as it can cause quicker browning.

4. **Stevia**: A highly concentrated sweetener derived from a plant. It's intensely sweet and doesn't add bulk, so use sparingly and adjust liquids.

5. **Erythritol**: A sugar alcohol that provides sweetness without impacting blood sugar levels. It measures like sugar but can have a cooling effect in large quantities.

Each substitute has unique properties that affect taste, texture, and baking properties, so choose based on your recipe and desired outcome.

Conversion Essentials

Converting recipes from sugar to substitutes requires precision. Use these conversion guidelines:

- **Honey**: Use 1/2 to 2/3 cup for every cup of sugar and reduce liquids by 1/4 cup for each cup of honey used.
- **Maple Syrup**: Replace 3/4 to 1 cup for every cup of sugar and reduce other liquids by 3 tablespoons per cup of syrup.
- **Agave Nectar**: Substitute 3/4 cup for every cup of sugar and decrease other liquids by 1/4 cup for each cup of agave used.
- **Stevia**: Follow manufacturer's guidelines as potency varies; usually, a small amount (1 teaspoon or less) can replace a cup of sugar.

For erythritol, use 1 1/4 cups for every cup of sugar and note it may affect texture and browning, so adjustments may be needed.

Adjusting Texture and Moisture

Maintaining the texture and moisture in baked goods:

- **Texture**: Substitute some sugar with moist ingredients like applesauce or yogurt to retain texture.
- **Moisture**: Increase liquids or add extra eggs to compensate for reduced moisture from sugar substitutes.

Flavor Enhancement

Enhance flavors when using substitutes:

- **Spices and extracts**: Add cinnamon, vanilla, or citrus zest to complement flavors.
- **Complementary ingredients**: Use nuts, dried fruits, or chocolate to balance and enhance taste profiles.

Baking Techniques

Effective techniques for baking with sugar substitutes:

- **Caramelization**: Adjust baking temperatures to prevent over-browning with substitutes like honey or maple syrup.
- **Mixing**: Modify mixing times to accommodate different textures and ingredients.

Health Considerations

Consider health factors when choosing substitutes:

- **Glycemic Index**: Opt for substitutes like stevia or erythritol for lower impacts on blood sugar levels.
- **Calorie Content**: Some substitutes offer fewer calories per serving compared to sugar, supporting weight management goals.

Sample Recipes

Try these adapted recipes to explore the versatility of sugar substitutes:

- **Vanilla Maple Cupcakes**: Replace sugar with maple syrup for a moist and flavorful treat.
- **Blueberry Lemon Muffins**: Use agave nectar for a lightly sweetened, tender muffin.
- **Homemade BBQ Sauce**: Sweeten with stevia for a lower-calorie, diabetic-friendly option.

FAQ Section

Common questions about substituting sugar:

- **Can I substitute any sweetener in any recipe?**

  Each sweetener behaves differently, so adjustments may be needed for best results.

- **How do I prevent my baked goods from becoming too dry?**

  Increase moisture with ingredients like applesauce or adjust baking times and temperatures.

- **Which sweetener is best for diabetic-friendly recipes?**

  Stevia or erythritol are typically good choices due to their minimal impact on blood sugar levels.

By mastering these tips and understanding the nuances of each sugar substitute, you can confidently adapt recipes to meet your dietary needs and preferences without sacrificing taste or quality. Experimentation is encouraged to find your perfect balance of sweetness in every dish!

Health Considerations

Weight Management and Sugar Substitutes

In the pursuit of healthier eating habits and managing weight, sugar substitutes have emerged as a viable alternative to traditional sugars. These substitutes promise the sweet taste we crave without the added calories, making them increasingly popular in modern dietary trends. Let's delve into the role of sugar substitutes, such as stevia, erythritol, and monk fruit, in weight management, examining their effectiveness, scientific insights, and practical integration into a balanced diet.

Effectiveness of Sugar Substitutes in Reducing Calorie Intake

1. Stevia: Derived from the leaves of the Stevia rebaudiana plant, stevia is known for its intense sweetness. It contains zero calories and has a negligible effect on blood glucose levels, making it suitable for diabetics and those watching their calorie intake. Studies have shown that stevia can help reduce overall calorie consumption by replacing high-calorie sweeteners in beverages and foods.

2. Erythritol: A sugar alcohol naturally found in fruits and fermented foods, erythritol provides sweetness with about 70% of the sweetness of sugar but with only 6% of the calories. It is absorbed into the bloodstream but largely excreted unchanged through urine, so it does not affect blood sugar or insulin levels. Erythritol is popular for its minimal impact on gastrointestinal tolerance compared to other sugar alcohols.

3. Monk Fruit: Monk fruit extract, derived from the monk fruit (Siraitia grosvenorii), is up to 250 times sweeter than sugar. It contains compounds called mogrosides that provide sweetness without calories. Monk fruit sweeteners do not raise blood sugar levels and are considered safe for individuals with diabetes. Like stevia and erythritol, monk fruit sweeteners offer a way to enjoy sweetness without the metabolic consequences of sugar.

Scientific Insights into Sugar Substitutes vs. Traditional Sugars

Traditional sugars like sucrose (table sugar) and high-fructose corn syrup contribute significantly to calorie intake without providing essential nutrients. Consuming excess sugars is linked to weight gain, obesity, and various metabolic disorders. In contrast, sugar substitutes provide sweetness without the calories, thereby reducing overall energy intake. They do not contribute to dental caries and do not cause the same rapid spike and crash in blood glucose levels as traditional sugars, making them preferable in managing weight and blood sugar levels.

Practical Tips for Integrating Sugar Substitutes into a Balanced Diet

To effectively integrate sugar substitutes into your diet for weight management:

- **Read Labels:** Look for products that use stevia, erythritol, or monk fruit as sweeteners instead of sugar.
- **Gradual Transition:** Start by replacing sugary beverages with those sweetened with substitutes.
- **Baking and Cooking:** Use sugar substitutes in recipes for baked goods and sauces, adjusting quantities to achieve desired sweetness.
- **Be Mindful of Other Sources:** Sugar substitutes are often combined with other ingredients in processed foods, so be aware of overall nutritional content.

Addressing Myths and Misconceptions

1. Cancer Risk: There is no scientific evidence linking stevia, erythritol, or monk fruit to cancer risk in humans.

2. Long-term Health Effects: Extensive research supports the safety of these sugar substitutes when consumed within acceptable daily intake levels.

3. Cravings and Appetite: While sugar substitutes provide sweetness, they do not trigger the same satiety responses as sugars. Moderation is key to managing cravings and appetite.

Dental Health: Sugar Substitutes and Your Teeth

Sugar substitutes have gained popularity not only for their potential health benefits in weight management but also for their role in preserving dental health. Understanding their impact on tooth decay, gum health, and overall oral hygiene is crucial in making informed dietary choices. Let's explore the comparative effects of popular substitutes like xylitol, sorbitol, and stevia on dental health, supported by insights from dental professionals and scientific research.

Comparative Effects of Sugar Substitutes on Tooth Decay and Gum Health

1. Xylitol: Widely recognized for its oral health benefits, xylitol is a sugar alcohol that cannot be fermented by oral bacteria like Streptococcus mutans, which are responsible for plaque formation and tooth decay. Studies have shown that regular consumption of xylitol can reduce levels of these harmful bacteria in the mouth, thereby decreasing the risk of cavities. Xylitol also promotes saliva production, which helps neutralize acids and remineralize enamel.

2. Sorbitol: Another sugar alcohol commonly used as a sweetener in sugar-free gums and candies, sorbitol is less effective than xylitol in preventing tooth decay. While it does not promote dental caries directly, sorbitol can still contribute to plaque formation if oral hygiene practices are inadequate.

3. Stevia: Unlike xylitol and sorbitol, stevia is a non-caloric sweetener derived from the leaves of the Stevia rebaudiana plant. It does not contribute to tooth decay because it is not metabolized by oral bacteria and does not ferment in the mouth. Stevia does not affect blood glucose levels, making it suitable for individuals with diabetes who are also concerned about dental health.

Insights from Dental Professionals and Scientific Studies

Dental professionals emphasize the importance of reducing sugar intake to maintain oral hygiene and prevent dental issues. Sugar substitutes offer a promising alternative by providing sweetness without the harmful effects of sugar on teeth. According to research published in the Journal of Dental Research, xylitol has been shown to significantly reduce the incidence of cavities when used regularly, especially in chewing gums and oral care products.

Practical Advice for Incorporating Sugar Substitutes into Daily Routines

To support dental hygiene while enjoying the benefits of sugar substitutes:

- **Choose Products Wisely:** Opt for chewing gums, mints, and oral care products sweetened with xylitol or stevia instead of sugar.
- **Maintain Oral Hygiene:** Brush teeth at least twice daily with fluoride toothpaste and floss regularly to remove plaque and food particles.
- **Moderate Consumption:** While sugar substitutes are beneficial, excessive consumption can still lead to gastrointestinal discomfort with sugar alcohols like xylitol and sorbitol.

Addressing Common Concerns and Misconceptions

1. Impact on Oral Microbiome: Sugar substitutes like xylitol do not disrupt the oral microbiome as sugars do, making them a safer option for dental health.

2. Long-term Effects: Extensive research supports the safety and efficacy of xylitol and stevia in promoting dental health when used as part of a balanced oral hygiene routine.

3. Taste and Acceptance: Advances in formulation have improved the taste and acceptance of products sweetened with sugar substitutes, making them more appealing to consumers.

Safety and Regulatory Considerations Sugar Substitutes

Sugar substitutes have become integral to modern dietary choices, offering sweetness with fewer calories and potential health benefits. However, ensuring their safety and regulation is crucial for consumer protection and informed decision-making. This article explores the regulatory considerations surrounding substitutes like stevia, erythritol, and monk fruit, delving into scientific evaluations, global regulatory frameworks, labeling practices, and emerging trends in safety research.

Regulatory Frameworks Governing Sugar Substitutes

1. Stevia: Stevia, derived from the Stevia rebaudiana plant, has gained global acceptance but faces varied regulations. In the United States, the FDA recognizes certain stevia extracts as Generally Recognized as Safe (GRAS) for use in food products. In the European Union (EU), steviol glycosides (the active compounds in stevia) are approved as food additives with established Acceptable Daily Intakes (ADIs).

2. Erythritol: As a sugar alcohol, erythritol is generally recognized as safe worldwide. It is approved as a food additive by regulatory bodies such as the FDA and the European Food

Safety Authority (EFSA). Erythritol's safety profile includes minimal impact on blood glucose and insulin levels, making it suitable for diabetics.

3. Monk Fruit: Monk fruit extract, known for its intense sweetness without calories, has been approved as a sweetener in various countries including the US, EU, and Australia. It is generally regarded as safe when used within recommended limits.

Scientific Basis for Evaluating Safety

The safety of sugar substitutes is assessed through rigorous scientific studies evaluating:

- **Toxicology:** Studies determine the potential for adverse effects such as genotoxicity, carcinogenicity, and reproductive toxicity.
- **Metabolism:** Research examines how substitutes are absorbed, metabolized, and excreted in the body, ensuring they do not accumulate or cause harm.
- **Health Impacts:** Long-term studies assess impacts on weight management, glycemic control, and overall health, comparing substitutes to traditional sugars.

Regulatory Approaches: Natural vs. Artificial Substitutes

Regulatory bodies differentiate between natural (like stevia and monk fruit) and artificial substitutes (like aspartame and saccharin). Natural substitutes often have simpler regulatory pathways due to perceived safety from botanical origins, whereas artificial substitutes undergo more stringent evaluations due to chemical synthesis concerns.

Labeling Practices and Consumer Choice

Product labeling plays a crucial role in transparency and consumer choice. Regulations mandate clear labeling of sugar substitutes to inform consumers of their presence and quantity in products. This allows individuals to make informed decisions based on dietary preferences, health considerations, and taste preferences.

Emerging Trends in Sugar Substitute Safety Research

Ongoing research focuses on:

- **Microbiome Impact:** Studying how substitutes affect gut microbiota and overall digestive health.
- **Neurological Effects:** Assessing potential impacts on brain function and cognitive health.

- **Environmental Impact:** Evaluating sustainability and ecological footprint of substitute production and use.

Regulatory Adaptation to New Scientific Findings

Regulatory bodies continually update guidelines based on new scientific data. For example, recent studies on gut health impacts may prompt adjustments in ADIs or labeling requirements. This ensures that regulations evolve with scientific understanding to protect consumer health and safety effectively.

Conclusion

Making Informed Choices for a Healthier Lifestyle

In our quest for healthier eating habits, sugar substitutes have emerged as valuable allies, offering sweetness without the guilt of excess calories and adverse health effects associated with traditional sugars. This article aims to empower you with knowledge on substitutes like stevia, erythritol, and monk fruit, exploring their benefits, considerations, and practical tips for integrating them into your daily diet.

Benefits of Sugar Substitutes

1. Reduced Caloric Intake: Sugar substitutes provide sweetness with minimal to no calories, making them ideal for those aiming to manage weight or reduce calorie consumption.

2. Blood Sugar Control: Unlike regular sugars, substitutes like stevia and erythritol do not cause spikes in blood glucose levels, making them suitable for individuals with diabetes or those monitoring their glycemic index.

3. Dental Health: Many substitutes, especially xylitol and erythritol, do not contribute to tooth decay and may even support dental health by reducing plaque formation.

4. Versatility in Cooking: Sugar substitutes can be used in cooking and baking to recreate favorite recipes with reduced sugar content, offering a healthier alternative without sacrificing taste.

Considerations When Choosing Sugar Substitutes

1. Taste Profile: Each substitute has a distinct taste profile. Experiment with different options to find one that suits your palate and complements your dishes.

2. Digestive Tolerance: Sugar alcohols like erythritol and xylitol may cause gastrointestinal discomfort in some individuals when consumed in large amounts. Start with small quantities to gauge tolerance.

3. Processing and Additives: Some commercially available substitutes may contain additives or fillers. Opt for products with minimal ingredients and avoid those with unnecessary additives.

Practical Tips for Incorporating Sugar Substitutes

1. Read Food Labels: Learn to identify hidden sugars in packaged foods by checking ingredient lists and looking for alternative sweeteners like stevia, erythritol, or monk fruit.

2. Substitute in Recipes: Use substitutes in cooking and baking by adjusting quantities to achieve desired sweetness levels. Replace sugar in recipes with equivalent amounts of substitutes or use conversion charts for guidance.

3. Balance Sweetness and Nutrition: Consult with a nutritionist or health expert to find a balance between satisfying your sweet tooth and meeting nutritional goals. They can offer personalized advice based on your health needs and preferences.

Addressing Common Myths and Misconceptions

1. Cancer Risk: Scientific evidence does not support claims that sugar substitutes like stevia or erythritol increase cancer risk. Regulatory bodies thoroughly evaluate safety before approving substitutes for food use.

2. Natural vs. Artificial: Natural substitutes like stevia and monk fruit are derived from plants, whereas artificial substitutes undergo chemical synthesis. Both types undergo rigorous safety evaluations before approval.

3. Taste and Acceptance: Advances in formulation have improved the taste and acceptance of sugar substitutes, making them more widely embraced in diverse culinary applications.

Taking Steps Towards Healthier Eating Habits

By embracing sugar substitutes, you can embark on a journey towards healthier eating habits without sacrificing sweetness or enjoyment. Whether you aim to manage weight, control blood sugar levels, or improve dental health, substitutes like stevia, erythritol, and monk fruit offer versatile options to support your goals. Empower yourself with knowledge, experiment with different substitutes, and consult with experts to tailor your choices to your unique health needs. Together, let's embrace the benefits of sugar substitutes and pave the way towards a balanced and fulfilling lifestyle.

Appendix

Glossary of Terms

1. Glycemic Index (GI): The glycemic index measures how quickly carbohydrates in a food raise blood sugar levels compared to pure glucose, which has a GI of 100. Foods with a low GI (55 or less) are digested and absorbed more slowly, causing a gradual rise in blood sugar levels. This is beneficial for maintaining stable energy levels and is often recommended for those managing diabetes or seeking to control their weight. For example, lentils have a low GI due to their high fiber content, which slows down digestion.

2. Stevia Rebaudiana: Stevia rebaudiana is a South American plant known for its intensely sweet leaves. Extracts from these leaves, such as steviol glycosides, are used as natural sweeteners. Stevia is non-caloric and does not affect blood sugar levels, making it a popular choice for people looking to reduce sugar intake. It is about 200 to 400 times sweeter than table sugar (sucrose). Stevia is commonly used in beverages, desserts, and as a tabletop sweetener.

3. Polyols (Sugar Alcohols): Polyols are a group of sugar substitutes that are partially absorbed by the body. They provide fewer calories than sugar and have a smaller impact on blood sugar levels, making them suitable for people with diabetes. Examples include erythritol, xylitol, and sorbitol. Polyols are used in sugar-free candies, chewing gums, and baked goods to provide sweetness and texture without the drawbacks of sugar.

4. Erythritol: Erythritol is a polyol that occurs naturally in fruits such as grapes and melons. It is about 70% as sweet as sugar but provides only about 0.2 calories per gram, compared to 4 calories per gram in sucrose. Erythritol does not raise blood sugar or insulin levels significantly and is well tolerated by most people when consumed in moderate amounts. It is commonly used in sugar-free chocolates, beverages, and baking recipes.

5. Xylitol: Xylitol is a sugar alcohol found in many fruits and vegetables. It has a sweetness similar to sugar and about 2.4 calories per gram. Xylitol has a minimal effect on blood sugar and insulin levels, making it suitable for diabetics. It also has dental benefits and is often used in chewing gums, mints, and oral care products to prevent tooth decay. However, excessive consumption may cause digestive issues in some individuals.

6. Sucralose: Sucralose is an artificial sweetener made from sugar. It is about 600 times sweeter than sugar but contributes negligible calories because it is not metabolized by the body. Sucralose is heat stable and can be used in cooking and baking. It is commonly found in diet sodas, sugar-free syrups, and processed foods as a sugar substitute. Unlike sugar alcohols, sucralose generally does not cause digestive upset.

7. Monk Fruit Extract (Luo Han Guo): Monk fruit extract is derived from the monk fruit, a small melon native to southern China. It is about 150 to 200 times sweeter than sugar but does not provide calories or raise blood sugar levels. Monk fruit extract contains antioxidants called mogrosides, which give it its intense sweetness. It is used in beverages, yogurts, and as a tabletop sweetener. Monk fruit extract has a clean, fruity taste and is well tolerated by most people.

8. Agave Nectar: Agave nectar is a natural sweetener derived from the sap of the agave plant, primarily grown in Mexico. It is about 1.5 times sweeter than sugar and has a low glycemic index, meaning it does not cause a rapid spike in blood sugar levels. Agave nectar is often used as a vegan alternative to honey and can be found in baking recipes, sauces, and beverages. However, it is still high in fructose and should be used in moderation.

9. Inulin: Inulin is a type of soluble fiber found in plants such as chicory root, onions, and garlic. It has a mildly sweet taste but does not significantly affect blood sugar levels because it is not fully digested by the body. Inulin is often used as a bulking agent and prebiotic fiber in sugar-free and low-calorie foods, promoting gut health by feeding beneficial bacteria in the intestines. It can be found in yogurt, cereal bars, and dietary supplements.

10. Maltitol: Maltitol is a sugar alcohol derived from maltose. It is about 90% as sweet as sugar and has about 2.1 calories per gram. Maltitol does have a significant effect on blood sugar levels, but it is lower than that of sucrose. Maltitol is used in sugar-free candies, chocolate, and baked goods to provide sweetness with fewer calories.

11. Raw honey: is honey that is unprocessed and unheated, harvested straight from the honeycomb. Unlike processed honey, which undergoes heating and filtration to remove impurities and delay crystallization, raw honey retains its natural properties and is not pasteurized

12. Maple syrup: is a natural sweetener derived from the sap of sugar maple trees (Acer saccharum).

13. Aspartame: A low-calorie artificial sweetener composed of aspartic acid and phenylalanine, commonly used in sugar-free and low-calorie food and beverage products.

14. Sucralose: is an artificial sweetener that is derived from sucrose (table sugar) through a chemical process that substitutes three chlorine atoms for three hydroxyl groups on the sugar molecule. This modification enhances its sweetness significantly—approximately 600 times sweeter than sucrose—while providing a negligible caloric contribution to the diet because it is not metabolized by the body for energy.

15. Saccharin: is an artificial sweetener that has been used for over a century as a sugar substitute. In summary, saccharin is valued for its intense sweetness, stability under various conditions, and role in providing low-calorie or sugar-free options for consumers. It has a long history of use and has been determined to be safe for most people when consumed within recommended levels.

16. Coconut sugar: also known as coconut palm sugar, is a natural sweetener derived from the sap of the coconut palm tree (Cocos nucifera). It is produced through a process of collecting the sap, heating it to evaporate the moisture, and then granulating it into sugar crystals. Coconut sugar retains some of the nutrients present in the coconut palm sap, including minerals such as iron, zinc, calcium, and potassium, as well as antioxidants and short-chain fatty acids.

17. Date sugar: is a natural sweetener made from dried, ground dates (Phoenix dactylifera), typically without any additional processing. Unlike other sugars, date sugar is not extracted from the fruit's sap but consists of finely ground whole dates. It retains the natural nutrients and fiber present in dates, making it a minimally processed alternative sweetener.

18. Yacon syrup: is a natural sweetener derived from the roots of the yacon plant (Smallanthus sonchifolius), native to the Andean regions of South America. The syrup is extracted from the tuberous roots of the plant and undergoes minimal processing to preserve its natural properties.

Resources for Further Reading

Books:

1. **The Complete Guide to Natural Sweeteners** by Alan Barclay and Philippa Sandall - Offers comprehensive insights into various natural sweeteners and their applications.
2. **Sweeteners: Nutritional Aspects, Applications, and Production Technology** edited by Ruth Smith - Provides a deep dive into the nutritional aspects and production technologies of sweeteners.

Websites and Online Resources:

1. **The Sugar Association** - Provides information on sugar substitutes and their impact on health.
2. **Mayo Clinic** - Offers a guide to artificial sweeteners, their safety, and impact on health.

Scientific Journals and Articles:

1. **Nutrients** - Publishes research articles on the health effects of various sweeteners and their nutritional profiles.

2. **Journal of the Academy of Nutrition and Dietetics** - Contains studies on glycemic index and nutritional aspects of alternative sweeteners.

Cookbooks and Recipes:

1. **Naturally Sweet: Bake All Your Favorites with 30% to 50% Less Sugar** by America's Test Kitchen - Features recipes that use alternative sweeteners while reducing sugar content.

2. **The Stevia Cookbook: Cooking with Nature's Calorie-Free Sweetener** by Ray Sahelian - Focuses on recipes using stevia, a natural sweetener.

Organizations and Associations:

1. **American Diabetes Association** - Provides resources on sugar substitutes and their role in diabetes management.

2. **International Food Information Council** - Offers information on food ingredients, including sweeteners, and their impact on health.

Blogs and Online Communities:

1. **Minimalist Baker** - Features recipes and tips for using alternative sweeteners in baking and cooking.
2. **Wellness Mama** - Offers articles and guides on healthy eating, including alternatives to refined sugars.

Documentaries and Educational Videos:

1. **Documentaries on the sugar industry** - Explore documentaries that discuss the sugar industry's impact on health and alternatives.
2. **Educational videos on YouTube** - Channels and videos discussing the science behind sugar substitutes and their benefits.

Ditya Zulkarnain